# Praise for
# *27 Things To Know About Yoga*

Victoria has written a wonderful book about the foundations of yoga practice explained in a way that is accessible, informative, and down-to-earth. Whether you are a yoga newbie who is learning the ropes or an experienced yogi who wants to get back to basics, you'll be inspired to roll out your mat and get started!

*—Nora Isaacs*
*Former senior editor at* Yoga Journal *magazine*
*and author of* Women in Overdrive: Find Balance and Overcome Burnout at Any Age

*27 Things* is the perfect book for anyone who is thinking about diving into the world of yoga. By providing in-depth information on the origins of yoga as well as many resources, *27 Things* demystifies the power of yoga while presenting a practical approach.

*—Tisha Morris*
*Author of* 27 Things To Feng Shui Your Home

Victoria is a friendly, funny, and knowledgeable guide to all things yoga. Her book can help you stop wondering about yoga and get inspired to start practicing it. Buy one copy for yourself, and one for your friend, family member, boyfriend, [or] girlfriend who needs a little help with starting a self-care practice.

*—Kate Hanley*
*Author of* The Anywhere, Anytime Chill Guide,
*and founder of* msmindbody.com

# 27 Things To Know About Yoga

This book is dedicated to my father, Harold Lee Everman, Jr. (7/23/57–3/22/06): you loved so passionately that it stopped your heart. I wish I could have introduced you to the beauty of yoga.

# 27 Things To Know About Yoga

Victoria Klein

Trade Paper
Press

Turner Publishing Company
200 4th Avenue North • Suite 950
Nashville, Tennessee 37219
(615) 255-2665

www.turnerpublishing.com

*27 Things To Know About Yoga*

Library of Congress Cataloging-in-Publication Data

Klein, Victoria, 1984-
 27 things to know about yoga / by Victoria Klein.
    p. cm.
 ISBN 978-1-59652-590-0
 1. Hatha yoga. I. Title. II. Title: Twenty-seven things to know about yoga.
 RA781.7.K58 2010
 613.7'046--dc22
                              2010015810


Printed in China

10 11 12 13 14 15 16 17—0 9 8 7 6 5 4 3 2 1

*Our life is shaped by our mind; we become what we think.*

—Buddha

# Contents

# Acknowledgements

# Acknowledgements

In all of life, one thing is constant: family. I wouldn't be here without them (literally!) and they deserve first mention. My beautiful mother, Beverly E.: you never cease to amaze me with your inner strength, personal resolve, and frank intelligence (what should we make next?). Sara G., my only sister: a soul as striking as yours deserves to shine; you've quietly supported me all these years and I just wouldn't be the same without you (you still have better hair than me). My stepdad, John L.: how you put up with all my teenage crap, I'll never know, but you remained sane through it all and introduced me to the grace that is Europe (*viva Italia!*). My Gram, Janice M.: a huge dose of my creativity and curiosity for nature originates with you, making my childhood better than I could have hoped for (national parks rock!).

A few special folks have come into my life and made my head spin, changing my perspective for the better. My husband, Logan K.: I never imagined my fifth-grade crush would change my life . . . and our vibrant journey has just begun (ooh-rah, but no kids yet). My best (male) friend, Matt B.: we've loved and lost and loved again; our paths continue to be intertwined and I wouldn't want it any other way (Buddhism dude). My best (female) friend, Shannon K.: all those cheeseburgers and orange sodas were a perfect accessory to our introspective chats, with many more to come—thank you (from Howie). My SF homie, Tess B.: your bear hugs and spunky charisma always make me smile (Ren Fair, tattoos, and scooters). The best neighbor ever, Lisa S.: you were my first "adult" friend, always inspiring me to push forward and live boldly (wives of the gamer guys).

My yoga journey has been touched by some spectacular people worth noting. My SF yoga studio, Yoga Tree: my managers, fellow employees, and the adorable Tim and Tara Dale helped me find firm footing on my exploration of yoga, both as an employee and a student (eighty students in fifteen minutes? I can handle that). My SF teachers, Catherine Chapman, K. K. Ledford, Janet Stone, Stephanie Snyder, and Jehfree Spirit: you all helped take my physical practice and internal voice to a level I couldn't attain on my own (always remember to breathe). The crew at *Yoga Journal,* Diane Anderson, Brian Castellani, Charity Ferreira, Claudia Smukler, and Jane Tarver: you all made my time at the magazine memorable, educational, and downright fun; keep the assignments coming (conference room + downward dog = best lunch hour ever).

My name may be on the cover, but these folks provided a vital contribution to this book's success. My acquisitions editor at Turner, Michael McCalip: you believed in me and I can never repay you for this chance (there's no such thing as too many questions). The dear yoga teachers who gave their time and knowledge—Frank Jude Boccio, Elena Brower, Les Leventhal, David Lurey, Jeanie Garden, Peter Guinosso, and Natasha Rizopoulos: your insights took this book from mediocre to awesome.

Without the many vibrant connections I've made on the Internet, my personal and professional life would be nothing like it is today. A *huge* thank you to all my buddies on Livejournal, Flickr, Facebook, Twitter, Etsy, and my blog: your comments brighten me daily. Special thanks to Tara Hogan, Susan Piver, and Nicole Hill Gerulat: the Web connected us, and working with each of you has been nothing short of pure joy (we'll meet in person someday, someday).

# Introduction

# Introduction

Your cousin, your best friend, that cute cashier at the grocery store: there's a good chance they all practice yoga. Unless you've been in a coma for the past decade, then you may have noticed the huge rise in yoga's popularity. By picking up this book, you've shown that you are ready to try this fantastic practice, and I applaud you. Welcome to the club!

Yoga is fun, affordable, and pressure-free. With yoga studios, DVDs, and books more prolific than ever, you can easily find a practice that is just right for you in every way. No matter your age, size, color, or occupation, you can benefit from the many gifts that yoga has to offer—physical strength, flexibility, stamina, mental clarity, patience, and countless health improvements (many of which I'll talk about later). Before beginning any physical routine, including the practice of yoga, you should consult a physician or other medical professional. Note: tan skin, blonde hair, and leotard not required.

Whether you've already started a new yoga practice or are an honest-to-goodness beginner, this book will give you a hearty introduction to all the basic aspects of yoga. Think of this as a gateway book, a great starting point or quick reference in your ongoing journey for intelligent and useful information about yoga. Still hesitant about delving into the wide world of yoga? Never fear—that's why I'm here!

This guide is here to help you make sense of all the yoga hype (some of which is total poppycock!). Read through the whole book in one afternoon or just skip to the section you are curious about. Put aside your preconceived notions and give yoga a chance to make a positive difference in your life. Then you'll see what all the fuss is about.

# The 27 Things

# ~ 1 ~

# Yoga: a definition

# ~ 1 ~

# Yoga: a definition

To start things off right, here are a few things yoga is not: a cult, a religion, an overnight sensation, hedonism, self-torture, or magic. The misconceptions about yoga are many, but the truth is very simple. Practicing yoga is about awareness and relationships, allowing us to become more in tune with our mental and emotional patterns.

Translated from Sanskrit, the word *yoga* means "union" or "to join together." Yoga is a combination of physical (poses and breathing) and mental (meditation) practices designed to help free us from our attachments to the material world, uniting our body and mind. "Classically speaking, yoga is the art and science of observing and calming the fluctuations of the mind to realize or inherent divine and interconnected nature," says David Lurey, certified yoga teacher, trainer, and cofounder of Green Yoga (GreenYoga.org; FindBalance.net). "The modern application of this has become a dynamic and powerful practice of the body, mind, and spirit that leads to the same realizations."

That may sound a bit hokey, but you can't practice the well-known *asanas* (poses) of yoga without concentrating; your mind and your body are forever connected. All it takes is one good yoga practice to change your outlook for days. Prepare to share the smiles: a happy body and mind brightens not only your day, but also the day of those around you.

While some may think it nothing more than a trend, yoga's physical practice and spiritual philosophies have been known in the United States since the 1890s, escalating in popularity from the 1960s to today. Even more impressive is that yoga itself is reputed to have been around for 5,000 years (give or take a few centuries). The *Rig Veda,* one of the oldest books ever written, contains distinct elements of yoga. Dating to sometime between 1500 B.C. and 900 B.C., the *Rig Veda* contains words that are believed to be many generations older than the book itself, passed down through a strong oral tradition.

The ultimate origins of yogic concepts are essentially unknown. They simply precede existing written record. A scholar named Patanjali wrote the first inclusive guide on the subject, titled the *Yoga Sutras*. The book is believed to have been written around 200 B.C. and contains the formal yoga philosophies taught today all over the world. A few other books are excellent examples of yogic beliefs (i.e., *Bhagavad Gita*), but Patanjali's *Sutras* was the first all about the practice of yoga. Numerous translations of the Sanskrit-scribed *Yoga Sutras* are available in bookstores, each with their own subtle differences in interpretation (see Thing 27 for recommendations).

Despite its many philosophical aspects, yoga today is widely known for its poses or postures, known in Sanskrit as *asanas*. Also called *hatha* yoga (see Thing 13), the physical practices of yoga were first recorded in-depth by Swatmararma Yogindra during the 1400s within the *Hatha Yoga Pradipika.* The overarching theme of his manual was to link the purification of both the body and the mind into one system. As with the *Yoga Sutras,* translations of the *Hatha Yoga Pradipika* are widely sold (see Thing 27).

As you can see, yoga has a long history of time-tested concepts for the body and mind. You don't have to change your religion or diet to embrace yoga, but it may inspire you to ask questions of yourself and the world in which you live.

## ~ 2 ~

# For one and for all!

# – 2 –

# For one and all!

Despite the yoga models you may see in magazines or on TV, yoga is for everyone. There's not one thing that can get in your way of practicing all the joys of yoga. Age, weight, sex, color, finances, flexibility, past injuries, handicaps—none of them can stop you. You do not have to be in tip-top, average, or even decent physical condition to practice yoga.

Oh, wait—there is one roadblock to overcome: your mind. If you think you can't do it, then you won't. No matter what you have heard or think you know about yoga, push it all out of your head and start anew. Each time you step onto the mat, you offer yourself the opportunity to grow in ways you never imagined.

To a newcomer, the world of yoga can seem a bit overwhelming. Among the choices to be made, selecting a yoga style or type is at the top of the list. Thankfully, this is a decision you can make many times with little regret. After taking a single class and then classes offering two to four different styles, you will quickly be able to identify which works best for your personality and physical abilities.

What can you expect? Though every style is different, yoga classes have an overall similar execution. First, you spend five to fifteen minutes getting mentally centered on the moment while sitting still and performing minor stretches. Next, you perform the majority of physical poses, starting with simpler, one-muscle-group poses before progressing to standing, full-body *asanas*. Third, you practice seated and supine (lying-down) poses. Last but never least, you enjoy *savasana* (corpse pose; see Thing 23) for five to fifteen minutes.

The following is a short, but by no means all-encompassing, overview of the most well-known and widely offered yoga styles. I've arranged the class styles in order of intensity to make selection easier. Use this information to assist you in choosing which classes to dabble in.

*Hatha:* A general term for all styles of posture-focused yoga practices, usually featuring an equal amount of physical exertion and relaxation.

**Gentle (little to no sweating with minor physical effort)**

*Ananda:* Developed by Swami Kriyananda in the 1960s. A gentle, classical style using internal affirmations during the physical practice to prepare for future meditation and personal exploration. (www. anandayoga.org)

*Prenatal:* A gentle class meant for pregnant women. Not based on any particular traditional style. Focus is placed on reducing aches, pains, and preparing the body and mind for childbirth.

*Restorative:* The name says it all: a therapeutic, gentle practice in which the body is supported by props, and poses are held for long periods of time. Often recommended once a week to complement a regular, more active yoga practice or for those with physical limitations.

*Sivananda:* Founded by Swami Vishnu-devananda in 1957 and named for his teacher Swami Sivananda. A gentle, introspective, beginner-friendly practice meant solely to benefit spiritual development. Twelve key poses, along with chanting and meditation, make up the classes. (www.sivananda.org)

*Viniyoga:* Created by T. K. B. Desikachar and introduced to the U.S. by Gary Kraftsow in 1999. A gentle form with particular focus placed on coordinating the breath with movement through poses. Excellent for beginners as poses and classes are customized based on each student's abilities, needs, and restrictions. (www.viniyoga.com)

## Active (some sweating and effort)

*Anusara:* Established by John Friend in 1997. Translates as "following the heart" and focuses on an "individually appropriate, alignment-centered, joy-filled practice." Each class usually focuses on a single theme that is reflected upon throughout. (www.anusara.com)

*Ashtanga:* Founded by K. Pattabhi Jois in the 1920s. Translated as "eight-limbed yoga" and based directly on Patanjali's *Yoga Sutras.* A physically demanding, uninterrupted practice centered on observing the self without attachment or analyzation. (www.ashtanga.com; www.kpjayi.org)

*Integral:* Founded in 1966 by Sri Swami Satchidananda. This is a combination of the many branches of yoga (see Thing 13), including the physical practice and beyond—more of a lifestyle than just a series of postures. Focus is placed on providing a practice for anyone and everyone, with modifications readily made. (www.yogaville.org; www.iyiny.org)

*Iyengar:* Established by B. K. S. Iyengar. Features a slower pace that focuses on promoting physical alignment and understanding how the body works. Props and adjustments are common, making this a safe option for many. Teachers are subjected to a rigorous two to five years of training before being certified. (www.bksiyengar.com; www.iynaus.org)

*Kripalu:* Established by Amrit Desai, a.k.a. Swami Kripalu, in 1966. Arranged in three stages of complexity, focus is put on proper physical alignment and breathing with encouragement of inquiry and natural curiosity both on and off the mat. (www.kripalu.org)

*YogaFit:* Founded by Beth Shaw in 1994. Short for "Yoga for the Fitness Industry" and meant to "introduce yoga to everyone, free of dogma." Often taught in gyms and fitness centers, expect a mix of yoga poses and traditional strength exercises, such as push-ups and sit-ups. (www.yogafit.com)

**Intense (lots of sweating and effort)**

*Bikram/Hot:* Introduced to the U.S. in 1971 by founder Bikram Choudhury. A set sequence of twenty-six poses performed in a humid room heated to at least 100 degrees Fahrenheit. The specific poses and high temps are meant to "clean the body from inside out." (www.bikramyoga.com)

*Forrest:* Created by Ana Forrest in 1982. Expect a strong, sweat-inducing practice meant to release physical and emotional tension. Particular focus is placed on the body's core (abs and back) to "help practitioners connect to their life's purpose." (www.forrestyoga.com)

*Jivamukti:* Founded by David Life and Sharon Gannon in 1984. Translated as "liberation while living." Expect a vivid practice combining physically challenging and mentally stimulating elements. An eclectic variety of music, chanting, and meditation are featured in each class. (www.jivamuktiyoga.com)

*Kundalini:* Founded by Yogi Bhajan in 1969. A vigorous practice including quick postures, challenging breathing exercises, meditation, and more. Focus is placed on self-awareness and personal transformation. (www.kriteachings.org; www.yogibhajan.com)

*Vinyasa/Power/Flow:* Known under many names, one factor remains constant—students flow from one pose to the next while synchronizing their poses and their breathing. Some classes are performed in a heated room (though not as hot as Bikram). Usually fast-paced, featuring a mix of traditional Indian and popular music. Better for students who have practiced for a few months and already understand the correct alignment of poses.

Still struggling to find the right style? Talk to a yoga teacher—they are the professionals, after all. Tell them about your personality, available time, and physical condition. With that information, any experienced yoga teacher should be able to give you a proper recommendation (and possibly the referral to teachers of that style).

# — 3 —

# Not a religion

# — 3 —

# Not a religion

A very dicey subject is the relationship between yoga and religion, but it is a valid concern among those contemplating a yoga practice. Christian, Jewish, Muslim, Buddhist, Hindu—anyone can practice yoga.

No, yoga is not a religion.

Yoga is a physical and mental practice, but it does not require deity worship, rituals, sacred icons, or membership (all elements that are part of the definition of religion). Being spiritual, yoga is centered on exploring the self and our place in the world. In comparison, religion is a counterpart to spirituality, focusing on an externalized organizational structure.

You will not be betraying your faith by chanting *om* or saying *namaste* to your teacher (see Thing

4 on Sanskrit words). One of the ultimate goals of yoga is liberation. Chanting is just another way of opening up the mind, but as with any other element of yoga, it is optional.

Everyone is welcome to their religious choice when practicing yoga. Still, there will be those who interpret yoga as a religion and, despite the given facts, will continue to believe so. In the end, those people are missing out on yoga's plentiful opportunities to grow in a myriad of ways. "Yoga provides us with an opportunity to pause and connect to our own divinity," says Elena Brower, certified yoga teacher for over twelve years and founder of New York's Virayoga studio (Virayoga.com). "Rather than something separate from ourselves, we're actually connecting to what is highest within ourselves."

Our world is full of numerous religions, each with their own explanations for the origin of our species and for our connection with what can't be seen. In a similar fashion, there is an ever-growing number of yoga styles, giving us the opportunity to select one that feels right for us and our religious path (see Thing 2). Whether you believe in one god, many gods, or no god at all, yoga is a spectacular extension of our search for understanding. "Many people find that yoga actually supports their existing religious tradition," says Natasha Rizopoulos, popular certified yoga teacher since 1997 (NatashaRizopoulos.com). "They discover that it helps them to integrate their spiritual beliefs into their daily activities in ways that are both tangible and profound."

The debate on whether yoga is a religion is vibrantly ongoing, with no end in sight. Just like the many religious texts, the concept of yoga is translated in many ways. When approaching the possibility of practicing yoga, I implore you to be open-minded. Don't let your fears or interpretations hold you back from trying yoga for yourself. "People of all faiths, beliefs, and religions can use the tools of a yogic life to deepen their spiritual practice," says David Lurey. "It's up to the practitioner to feel the essence of yoga's messages and apply them to their own beliefs."

If you are so inclined, delve into the wide world of written yogic knowledge, exploring the subject on your own terms. As with any other resource, yoga teachers are a fantastic asset in your search for understanding yoga's spirituality. Yoga is based on the concept that personal experiences and realizations trump untested theories. So don't be afraid to ask questions!

# ～ 4 ～
# Learning basic Sanskrit words

# − 4 −

# Learning basic Sanskrit words

When Patanjali wrote the *Yoga Sutras* in 200 B.C., the tome was recorded in Sanskrit. Now one of the twenty-two official languages of India, Sanskrit was as popular in B.C. Asian countries as Latin and Greek were in Europe. Today, you will hear several Sanskrit words in yoga class. Many yoga teachers choose to use the Sanskrit names of yoga poses but often use the English translations concurrently (no need for memorizing!). Here are a few of the most common Sanskrit words you will hear during your yoga experience, along with their English definitions. Sanskrit is pronounced phonetically, so if you find a word you are unsure of, just talk it out syllable by syllable.

*Asana* [ah-suh-nuh]: A physical posture or pose; the third limb of Patanjali's eight-limbed path of yoga (see Thing 14).

*Savasana* [sav-asana]: Corpse pose

*Trikoasana* [triko-asana]: Triangle pose

*Vrksasana* [vrks-asana]: Tree pose

*Bhakti* [buhk-tee]: Love or devotion; can be directed toward yourself, your teacher, family, strangers, or a divine being.

*Chakra* [chuhk-ruh]: Literally translated as "wheel"; metaphorically, it represents the centers of subtle energy within the body, each of which corresponds to a certain set of organs or ailments. The locations are at the base of the spine, genitals, navel, heart, throat, middle of the forehead, and top of the head.

*Dharma* [dahr-muh]: Duty, justice, character, merit, virtue, or righteousness.

*Guru* [goo-roo]: A spiritual teacher.

*Karma* [kahr-muh]: A principle of action based on the concept of cause and effect; the action, effects, and consequences of all our chosen actions.

*Mantra* [mahn-truh]: A sacred thought, prayer, or sound that can have a steadying effect on the mind via verbal recitation; often used as preparation for meditation.

*Mudra* [muh-drah]: A symbolic physical gesture often made with the hands; meant to maintain the circulation of *prana* (vital energy) within the body.

*Namaste* [nuhm-uh-stey]: A greeting or salutation, directly translated as "The light/Divine within me honors the light/Divine within you," in a spiritual, not religious, sense (see Thing 3).

*Om/Ohm/Aum* [awm]: Known as "the original mantra"; the most powerful and sacred sound from which all other mantras result.

*Prana* [prah-nuh]: The unseen vital energy or life force that flows through everyone and everything.

*Pranayama* [prah-nuh-ya-muh]: Conscious, controlled breathing that balances the *prana* within the body.

*Shanti* [shahn-tee]: Peace.

*Vinyasa* [vin-ya-sa]: A flowing sequence of yoga poses linked with the breath; often labeled as a specific yoga style (see Thing 2).

# ~ 5 ~

# Achieving benefits galore

# – 5 –

# Achieving benefits galore

Can yoga help you live a healthier life? You better believe it! Medical studies are beginning to prove the many constructive benefits of yoga that experienced teachers and students have long heralded. "All of yoga's medical benefits are a result of a heightened sense of self-awareness," says David Lurey. "They all require discipline and dedication to reach them."

## Asthma

The American College of Sports Medicine found a 43 percent improvement in patients' symptoms after ten weeks of yoga practice. Yoga's emphasis on posture and deep, lengthened breaths improves lung capacity, efficiency, and overall airflow, which can reduce the frequency and severity of asthmatic attacks.

## Arthritis

The slow, controlled movements of a yoga practice have been shown to decrease chronic pain and joint swelling in both osteoarthritis and rheumatoid arthritis sufferers at Johns Hopkins Arthritis Center.

## Back pain

A study at the West Virginia University School of Medicine found that, after practicing yoga for three months, people reported 70 percent less lower-back pain, and 88 percent of them reduced or stopped taking pain medication. Alignment and body awareness during yoga practice has been shown to reduce numerous types of acute and chronic back pain, including scoliosis, sciatica, and herniated discs.

## Blood pressure

Yale School of Medicine found "significantly reduced" systolic and diastolic blood pressure levels in hypertension patients who practiced yoga and meditation therapies—results that were comparable to drug therapy. Increased circulation and oxygenation of the blood are important outcomes of a continuous yoga practice.

## Cancer

While there is still no cure for cancer, yoga has been shown to reduce physical symptoms, mental stress, treatment side effects, and quality of life in both sufferers and survivors. Studies dating back as far as 1962 have proven the benefits of complementary stress-reduction therapies like yoga for many types of cancer. Significant results include regained strength, nausea reduction, and a rise in red blood cells.

## Depression and anxiety

Boston University's School of Medicine discovered a 27 percent increase of the neurotransmitter GABA within the brain after just one sixty-minute yoga practice. Low levels of GABA have been tied to anxiety, depression, and Alzheimer's. Yoga's mood-enhancing benefits are similar to those for asthma—slowing the breath and heart rate to reduce the body's stress response.

## Diabetes

Along with its stress-reduction and strength-building benefits, yoga may help reduce and manage glucose, while possibly encouraging insulin production, especially for those with Type 2 diabetes. Medical studies from India, Nepal, and Canada have all found similar benefits for those with diabetes who maintain a regular yoga routine.

## Flexibility

This may seem obvious, but no matter your range of motion, yoga can improve it. You won't see benefits after just one class, but sticking to a regular practice helps release the lactic acid built up in your muscles. This natural acid is what causes stiffness, tension, and pain. Along with the muscles, the body's soft tissues (tendons and ligaments) are stretched and massaged during yoga, helping you see greater overall flexibility.

## Insomnia

Regular physical activity has been proven to improve sleep, and yoga is no exception. Calming for both the body and the mind, restorative yoga poses are often recommended for those finding it difficult to fall or stay asleep. A small study on yoga practitioners at Harvard Medical School's Brigham and Women's Hospital found "statistically significant improvements" in all aspects of falling, staying, and awaking from sleep.

## Memory and concentration

Yoga and meditation have been proven to increase concentration, motivation, and memory in as little as eight weeks, thanks to a rise in blood circulation to the brain and overall stress reduction. These benefits extend to help ward off the effects or advancement of Alzheimer's.

## Menopause

Studies at both the University of Washington and the University of Pittsburgh have produced the same results: yoga can significantly reduce the frequency and severity of hot flashes for women in all stages of menopause. In turn, yoga may reduce the need for hormone replacement therapy and strengthen the body against future osteoporosis.

## Nutrition

The *Journal of the American Dietetic Association* reported a unique connection between a regular yoga practice and eating healthier. Yoga is believed to increase mindful eating: being aware of why you eat and when to stop. Curiously, the results indicated that no other type of physical activity produced the same mindful eating effects.

## Posture

Thanks to increased flexibility and strength from practicing yoga, your posture naturally improves. Development of the body's core muscles and general self-awareness are key slump-defying benefits of yoga. Good upright posture is directly connected to positive increases in heart, lung, spine, and digestive functions.

## Sexuality

Do yoga—your love life will thank you. With better control over your mind and body, you can truly relax and enjoy your more intimate encounters. Along with your new awareness, you may possess increased self-confidence, sensuality, and physical energy—your turn to take control!

## Stress

One of the top reasons many seek out yoga is to relax, and for good cause. Deep breathing and conscious focus during your practice help bring you into the moment, thereby quieting the mind and releasing unnecessary tension from your body. Both yoga and meditation have proven in countless studies to be potent forces against the many stresses that bombard us in modern society, pulling us out of the primitive fight-or-flight mentality.

And this is just the tip of the iceberg. No matter your physical or mental capacities, there is surely a benefit to adding a yoga practice into your life. "The greatest benefit yoga can offer is how to live a full, rich, joy-filled, compassionate life in the face of reality," says Frank Jude Boccio, certified yoga teacher and author of *Mindfulness Yoga: The Awakened Union of the Breath, Body, and Mind* (MindfulnessYoga.net). "Yoga offers freedom from fear."

# ~ 6 ~

# Keeping it pain-free

# − 6 −

# Keeping it pain-free

Yoga shouldn't hurt—but it can. Like any other physical activity, yoga comes with a risk of injury. You've probably heard that yoga can relieve many types of physical pain, and it can. Concurrently, with all the stretching, twisting, and breathing you'll be doing, you have to listen to your body and stop pushing when it tells you to.

The most common yoga injuries have two main causes:

1. *Inexperienced teachers:* Yoga teacher training is informally regulated (see Thing 26), and although most studios and gyms require teachers to have over 500 hours of yoga study, instructors don't need a special degree. Taking the time to find a teacher that you

feel comfortable with is just as important as picking a yoga style that is right for your body and personality (see Thing 2).

Many yoga studios and gym Web sites feature teacher profiles, including a history of their training. If you can't find this info, ask the teacher directly. This is your health we are talking about. If they have nothing to hide, teachers will be more than happy to talk about the time they've spent honing their profession.

2. *Foolhardy students:* "No pain, no gain" does *not* apply to yoga. Before class, you need to inform your teacher of any past injuries or current issues you are experiencing (including menstruation or medications you are taking). He or she will be able to appropriately coach you during class to make adjustments and prevent injury. While you're at it, grab some props. Most yoga studios and gyms have straps, blocks, bolsters, and blankets (see Thing 7) available to students. "Props help correct spinal alignment,

facilitate proper stretching, take undue stress off the joints, and support tight muscles so they can release," says David Lurey.

Yoga is a practice for your body and your mind. To make your yoga practice both safe and effective, you need to quiet your mind and listen to your body. The most common yoga injuries occur in five key areas: wrists, shoulders, lower back, knees, and the sacrum (the triangular bone at the base of your spine and center of your pelvis). Consciously pay attention to these areas during your practice; they tend to speak loudly. If you feel a pinch, strain, pop, or anything unusual, slowly come out of the pose. Quietly signal the teacher and tell her what you felt. She will let you know whether you need to make adjustments in the pose, use additional props, or avoid the session all together.

"There is a clear distinction between pain and sensation," says Lurey. "Pain is hot . . . and should be avoided at all measures. Sensation is usually dull and achy and yogis should go in search of this!"

Though it may seem unnecessary, it bears saying: yoga is not a competition. Everyone has their own level of flexibility. Comparing yourself to the lady or gentleman on the next mat is utterly pointless. This leads to nothing but frustration and injury, defeating the point of practicing yoga entirely. Make sure to tell that annoying voice in your head to shut his trap too—competing with yourself is just as dangerous.

"A yogi should learn how to discern discomfort and the 'pain of change' from the potential pain of injury," says yoga instructor Frank Jude Boccio. "The yogi is practicing to overcome the biggest addiction of all: self-centeredness or what Patanjali called *asmita:* the sense of 'I-am-ness.' This humili-ation of the ego is going to be painful! It's the pain of change, analogous to the pain one may feel when tissues are healing."

Because of these two significant causes of minor to major injury, I always recommend beginners start their yoga practice under the supervision of a profes-sionally trained teacher. It is also recommended that beginners seek out medical advice from a physician. After a few months, when you are physically aware of appropriate alignment in most poses, you can begin practicing in your own home as well.

# ~ 7 ~
# Using simple supplies

# – 7 –

# Using simple supplies

Like any other physical practice, yoga requires a few tools to get started. Although some of these supplies are not needed for every session or style, I encourage you to try them all; many items I never thought I would use turned out to be my favorites.

## 1. Yoga mat*

You should never practice yoga without a yoga mat (a.k.a. sticky mat). It will help you maintain balance and proper alignment, thanks to its distinctive texture. Mats come in a wide variety of colors, lengths, and prices. The concept of "you get you pay for" often applies to yoga mats.

It's better to invest in a thick, sustainably made mat that will last for many years. Cheaper mats are often made from PVC, a type of plastic made from petroleum, so for a greener choice, look for mats made from natural or recycled rubber (avoid if you are allergic), jute, and wood pulp (they're splinter-free). My favorite mat is made by eco-committed Jade Yoga (Jadeyoga.com). I've had my Jade mat for over five years and it's still going strong.

*Note:* Yoga mats need to be cleaned. There are numerous ways to do this, but here is an easy, affordable, sustainable method that won't damage your mat in the process (unlike putting it in a washing machine).

*Supplies:*
Medium-sized spray bottle
Water
Tea tree essential oil
A scented essential oil of your preference.
Suggestions: chamomile, eucalyptus, geranium,

grapefruit, lavender, lemongrass, peppermint, or rose. (MountainRoseHerbs.com)

*Directions:*
- Fill the spray bottle with water.
- Add eight drops of tea tree oil and eight drops of your chosen essential oil for scent.
- Attach spray nozzle to bottle and shake.
- Spray your mat, front and back, until lightly moistened.
- Hang to dry.

*Note #2:* Once your mat has been worn down and lost its texture, don't just throw it in the trash. Recycle it! Oodles of yoga studios and retailers accept old mats to be used with nonprofit groups or to physically recycle, turning them into brand-new mats. Visit RecycleYourMat.com for more information.

## 2. Strap*#

Often made from cotton or hemp, a strap is used to attempt and maintain poses that involve reaching your hands to your feet.

## 3. Block*

A block also helps you attempt and maintain poses you may not normally be able to do, usually those that involve reaching your hands to the floor. You'll find blocks made from foam, cork (my favorite), bamboo, and other types of sustainable wood.

## 4. Blanket*#

Any blanket, whether one or many, can be folded and used to take pressure off your knees or hips during poses or seated meditation. During *savasana* (corpse pose, see Thing 23), covering up with a blanket keeps your muscles warm and relaxed.

I recommend blankets made from organic cotton, wool, recycled fibers, or even some you already own (nothing is greener than that!). Be sure to choose a fabric that will not irritate your skin.

## 5. Bolster*#

Commonly available in two shapes, cylindrical or a flat rectangle, bolsters support your body during reclining poses. Thanks to the extra support, your muscles and tendons can relax and repair themselves more effectively. When you buy a brand-new bolster, it will be very firm, but the filling will settle with use. Look for bolsters with removable, washable covers, commonly made from cotton or linen.

## 6. Eye pillow*#

Another helpful tool during *savasana,* an eye pillow blocks out all light and puts gentle pressure on your eyes, helping to relieve tension. Many are made from soft fabrics, like silk or cotton, filled with lightweight seeds or grains (flax, cassia) and scented buds or leaves (lavender, peppermint).

*Mat and prop sources:* BareFootYoga.com, Kulae.com, Manduka.com, Gaiam.com, JadeYoga.com, WaiLana.com, HuggerMugger.com, YogaAccessories.com, YogaDirect.com.

## 7. Fitted clothing#

Though you may be a bit self-conscious, wearing fitted, stretchy clothing during yoga has a key purpose: alignment. If you are wearing loose clothing, your teacher won't be able to see how you are placed within a pose. This means you could end up sustaining injuries or learning improper alignment, neither of which are good. Of course, I highly encourage you to find clothing that is soft, comfortable, and easy to move in, but err on the side of caution and use fitted items.

- *Men and women:* BePresent.com, Prana.com, InnerWaves.org, KayaYogaWear.Etsy.com, LuluLemon.com, ShaktiActivewear.com, TheYCatalog.com.
- *Women only:* HardTailForever.com, Lucy.com, Athleta.com, Omnitom.com, Zobha.com, MarieWright.com.

## 8. An open mind

This is the one accessory you can't buy. Practicing yoga is a journey, not a destination. You will hear, see, and feel things you never imagined. You will grow in ways you couldn't previously perceive. The key is to just let it all happen. Don't stand in the way of your own happiness. Explore all your opportunities and leave the judging to the Olympics.

*\* Your local yoga studio may have these items available for students to use at little to no cost. Nearly every studio offers yoga mats on loan, though they cost*

*anywhere from $1–$5 per use. Other props are often available in each studio space for you to gather as needed before class begins.*

*# If you happen to be crafty (or know someone who is), you can make these props and supplies yourself!*

My advice is to make active use of all the props available at your local yoga studio of choice. Then, when you begin your accompanying at-home practice, you will know how to use these props appropriately and which props are worth investing in.

# — 8 —

# Remembering safety first

# − 8 −

# Remembering safety first

Although everyone should be conscious of how their body feels while practicing yoga (see Thing 6), those with certain medical condition or injuries need to take extra care. Make sure to spend a few minutes before class with your yoga teacher, informing her of your personal afflictions.

As with any physical practice, you should consult your doctor before taking yoga classes, especially when you have one of the conditions discussed in the following pages. My guidelines here are very general, and only a trained yoga teacher can customize postures for your current symptoms. However, you should always listen to your own body; if it feels uncomfortable, stop doing what you're doing, despite anyone's recommendation.

"Move mindfully and don't do something that hurts just to follow the rest of the class," says Jeanie Garden, certified yoga teacher for over ten years (JeanieYoga.com). "You know your body best and you're the one who feels it when it hurts. Most of all, enjoy yourself—the body responds well to a happy mind."

*Arthritis or carpal tunnel syndrome:* Poses that emphasis alignment and upright posture have been shown to reduce CTS and arthritis symptoms. That said, poses that put anywhere from half to all of your body weight on your wrists should be approached with caution. A common adjustment for balancing postures is to balance on your fists instead of open palms. Stretching the upper back, neck, shoulders, arms, hands, and wrists should be the main focus of your regular practice.

*Back pain or injury:* Poses that involve arching or twisting the torso should be approached with caution. If your doctor has advised you of any movements you should avoid all together, inform your teacher ASAP, and he will adjust the practice for you. For back-pain sufferers, it's better to start with less intense classes, working up to heated or flowing yoga styles if and when your symptoms subside.

*Heart problems:* For heart-disease or heart-attack sufferers, yoga's stress-reducing capabilities can help to improve symptoms and prevent dangerous recurrences. It is recommended that those with heart troubles avoid more intense, heated classes in the beginning, due to the challenging cardiovascular element. Inverted poses and complex breathing techniques should be approached with caution.

*High blood pressure:* Also called hypertension, those with HBP can safely practice forward bending, sitting, and lying-down postures. Backbending, twisting, or inverted postures should be approached with caution though not avoided entirely; they naturally increase blood pressure. If you are on medication that regulates your blood pressure, nearly all poses are open to you.

*Knee pain or injury:* Misalignment is the most common cause for knee-injury aggravation during yoga practice. When poses are aligned properly, yoga can actually increase the strength of the knee joints. Nearly any posture that involves bending the knees should be approached with caution. Straight-legged postures can help stretch the muscles along the front, back, and sides of the knee, but make sure not to hyperextend the knee.

*Menstruation:* Inversions or any pose that raises the groin above the heart should be avoided entirely during your period. These types of poses lend to the reversal of the physical "flow." All other poses can be practiced with no restrictions. Forward bends, twists, and backbends can be especially beneficial for reducing PMS and cramps.

*Neck pain or injury:* Nearly any pose that involves twisting or putting direct pressure on the neck can be adjusted, usually by simply keeping the neck stationary or supporting it with props. Correct posture and alignment are key to reducing symptoms and the possibility of further strain.

*Pregnancy:* A consistent prenatal yoga practice has been shown to reduce physical strain and even produce a smoother birthing experience. Yoga can be practiced throughout your entire pregnancy, though pose recommendations and cautions change with each trimester. The risk of dehydration and fatigue during yoga are greater when pregnant, so take extra precautions to move slowly and hydrate often. Whether you are a new or more established yoga practitioner, you should fully discuss your pregnancy with your chosen yoga teacher. Many studios offer prenatal-specific classes, and I highly recommend them for your entire pregnancy. After at least a month of in-studio classes, practicing with prenatal yoga DVDs at home is usually safe. Many teachers recommend that before returning to your yoga practice, wait until at least one month after you give birth, or longer if you have had a C-section.

# ‒ 9 ‒

# You are what you eat

# — 9 —

# You are what you eat

Let's get one of the biggest misconceptions out of the way: you do not have to be a vegetarian or vegan to practice yoga.

That being said, there is a very good chance you'll think twice about what you choose to consume when you follow a regular yoga routine. In a landmark study, the *Journal of the American Dietetic Association* has reported that practicing yoga leads to "mindful eating." This is the first medical proof that yoga can and does help people lose weight. Remarkably, the same mindful eating effect was not seen in other forms of physical activity like running or strength training.

In general, yoga's emphasis on calming the mind and appreciating the body can lead you to reconsider that chocolate bar and reach for an apple instead.

A vital part of yogic philosophy is the concept of *ahimsa* or non-harming (see Thing 15). We all know that lying, cheating, stealing, fighting, and killing hurt others, but many have also extended *ahimsa* to include the "harming" of raising animals for food.

Eating animal products is a very controversial and personal subject. I'm not here to tell you what is "right" or "wrong," but I will say that yoga's focus on purifying the body for meditation and spiritual understanding lends itself to eating more fruits, vegetables, and whole grains over anything you'd find at a fast-food joint.

"You will naturally want to eat more healthy because you begin to notice how non-healthy food feels in the body," says Peter Guinosso, certified yoga teacher with decades of additional fitness experience (YogaIsLife.net). "This process should be organic and not determined by other people's philosophy or food preferences." I can speak from personal experience and say that I crave much less sugar and meat than I did before beginning my yoga practice—though I still love to bake cookies and enjoy the occasional cheeseburger.

"Find what works for you; every body is different," says Les Leventhal, certified yoga teacher since 2005 (YogaWithLes.com). "Steer clear of people who command and demand that you must eat this or that. Don't just wing it because some yoga teacher said you must do this or else."

Concurrently, your yoga practice will be enhanced by eating a more sustainable array of foods that have had little to no mechanical processing. If you feel self-conscious in the kitchen, now is the time to grab a recipe and give it a try. Don't let fear hold you back from feeding your body what it naturally needs and wants. Still spooked? Try taking a cooking class at a local community college or house of worship, either alone or with friends.

A desire to eat healthier is just one of yoga's many unexpected benefits. For many, the shift is unconscious at first. Seek out foods that make you feel lighter and brighter, both inside and out. Use your newfound personal awareness to sit and be absorbed by each meal you have (a key element of mindful eating). Eating is not just another task on your to-do list; it is one of the most vital elements of your life that shouldn't always be delegated to someone else. Just like your yoga practice, your diet will transform in ways you never imagined—but that's all part of the fun.

# ~ 10 ~

# The teacher makes the student

# – 10 –

# The teacher makes the student

Choosing a yoga instructor is akin to seeking out a new dentist, hairstylist, or auto garage mechanic. It's not a decision you want to make without doing a bit of researching and asking around for opinions. You're entrusting your physical well-being to the hands of someone you barely know. When you're ready to seek out a qualified yoga teacher, there are only two resources you need to use:

1. *Friends and family:* There's nothing better than a personal recommendation from someone you know. Ask around and you just may be surprised at how many folks you know practice yoga.

2. *The Internet:* Specifically, visit the Yoga Alliance Web site (www.yogaalliance.org) and the Yoga Journal Directory (www.yogajournal.com/directory). At both of these expansive directories, you can search for registered yoga teachers by location, yoga style, or name.

After you've selected a few yoga teachers or studios that you'd be interested in, it's time to start making some phone calls. You could skip this step, but you run the risk of wasting money on a class that you may not end up enjoying or, even worse, possibly getting injured. "It's like a job interview—look at many candidates," says Les Leventhal. "You will know the right one when they come along, and the good news is that it won't be that one teacher forever."

A great yoga teacher will have the following qualifications:

1. *Registered Yoga Teacher (RYT):* Teachers registered with the Yoga Alliance, a nonprofit dedicated

to maintaining teaching standards, have had at least 200 hours of professional certified training. This official designation is a strong symbol of their technical experience and commitment. As with any other business, you can request to see his or her certification, and the instructor should be happy to share it with you.

2. *Specific yoga style:* Each teacher should be trained in one distinct style (see Thing 2); choose the instructor according to the style that you already know you want to practice. Ask each teacher to describe his own classes and the kind of students who usually attend. Does he have a Web site? How long has he been personally practicing yoga? These questions can be asked over the phone or in person, but I recommend a face-to-face conversation in order to get a real "feel" or understanding for each teacher.

If you feel comfortable with a teacher already, inquire about his class schedule and sign up for a spot

ASAP. I recommended taking classes with at least three different teachers before deciding who you'd like to practice with regularly. Not the right one? At the end of class, politely tell him that the experience doesn't meet your needs and ask if he can refer you to a teacher with an easier or more challenging class. "Keep trying teachers until you are uplifted and inspired," says Elena Brower, yoga teacher and Virayoga studio founder. "The teacher should guide you to your own experience, not force-feed you his or her experience."

A great yoga teacher will also have the following qualities:

1. *Welcoming:* At the beginning of class, you should feel happy to be there and be embraced with open arms (literally or figuratively). This is the teacher's passion and livelihood. Every student is important, and a great yoga teacher should make you feel that way. "The primary focus of yoga teachers is to cre-

ate an environment of safety where students are guided into sensation and away from pain with total awareness," says David Lurey.

2. *Compassionate:* When you join any new yoga class, discussing your injuries or limitations with the teacher is essential. A great yoga teacher should be focused 100 percent on you during this conversation, listening intently. This is your first chance to connect with the teacher as he or she should be genuinely concerned about your needs or worries.

3. *Respectful:* During both your personal conversation and throughout the class, the teacher should be conscious of your privacy and comfort level. Some people naturally feel shy about revealing medical woes or the fact that they are struggling in a particular pose. A great teacher will be understanding of your reserve and do her best to accommodate you.

4. *Informative:* Don't know Sanskrit? Never prac-

ticed yoga? That's okay—a great yoga teacher will tell you the English names of yoga poses, their physical benefits, how to execute them correctly, and alternative poses or adjustments for people with medical conditions or tight muscles. If you're unsure of your alignment or a strange sensation you're feeling, quietly get the teacher's attention. She should happily come over and assist you.

5. *Thankful:* Ninety minutes later and class is over. A great yoga teacher will thank everyone for coming and often wish you a wonderful rest of the day. This is another chance to connect with him or her, sharing how you felt about the class and whether it met your personal needs. Don't be afraid to be honest—again, helping others learn yoga is the teacher's business, and direct feedback is pure gold.

# ~ 11 ~

# Minding your manners

# — 11 —

# Minding your manners

A little consideration goes a long way. When taking your first yoga class, you may not be aware of the subtle decorum. Following these guidelines will ensure that you, your fellow students, and the all-important teacher will thoroughly enjoy your time spent together.

1. *Arrive early:* Make it a habit to arrive at least ten minutes before class. This will give you ample time to check in with the studio's front desk, store your belongings, and calm your mind for the upcoming practice. If you arrive less than five minutes late, enter the class and roll your mat out quietly while not chatting with students. More than five minutes late? Respect the teacher and the other students by taking

a different class. "Respecting other people means not making then wait, or distributing their practice by arriving late," says Frank Jude Boccio. "Think of it as an act of consideration and generosity to arrive at the studio early."

2. *Stay home when sick:* Yoga is practiced in close quarters, making it very easy for those around you to catch the bug you've got. Stay home, get some rest, and return to your favorite studio when your symptoms have subsided. This doesn't mean that you needn't practice yoga at all. Basic seating or lying posture can be performed at home while battling a cold. Hit with the flu? Give your mind and body a break—that's what it is asking for.

3. *Have an empty stomach:* Don't eat, drink alcohol, or smoke for at least two hours before class. The considerable amount of movement during yoga can disrupt digestion. If you need some extra energy,

snacking on a piece of fruit is best. Don't bring any food into class, but bringing a bottle of water is a-okay.

4. *Wear light (or no) perfumes or colognes:* If you sweat during your practice, any scents you are wearing will be intensified, which can be distracting to some and allergy-aggravating to others. Abstain from applying any perfumes, oils, or lotions before class. Save them for the shower after your session.

5. *Remove jewelry:* Similar to scented products, wearing jewelry during class can be distracting, both visually and audibly, for students and teachers alike. Please be considerate and remove your adornments before class.

6. *No shoes, no cell phone, no worries:* There are three key things to leave outside of the practice room. 1) Your shoes: remove your shoes right when you enter the yoga studio. 2) Your cell phone: turn

off your phone and leave it with your shoes outside of the classroom. 3) Your troubles: arriving early for class will ensure you have time to calm your mind and set your worries aside while you take care of yourself for the next ninety minutes.

7. *Bring your supplies:* Come prepared to practice by wearing (or changing into) fitted, comfortable clothing while toting your yoga mat and any other props you have (see Thing 7). If you plan to use props provided by the yoga studio, find a place for your mat and then collect everything you may need before the class begins.

8. *Respect the space of others:* Don't move another student's mat in order to roll out your own mat. Just pick another area in class. If there is no more space, you have two options: politely ask if a student could slide his or her mat over, or take a different class. Try arriving a few minutes earlier to your next class, allowing you ample time to find a space. Before rolling

out your mat, be sure that you are giving yourself and those around you enough room to practice. The general rule is to allow at least one foot between your mat and your neighbor's mat, though this may not always be possible in more popular classes.

9. *Talk with the teacher:* Before class starts, be sure to approach your yoga teacher and share any medical issues or chronic conditions you suffer from. This information is important to instructors, assisting in their ability to guard you against injury during the practice.

10. *Respect the teacher:* She is your guide to the world of yoga. Listen intently and follow all of your teacher's instructions. If something feels uncomfortable, quietly raise your hand or get her attention for help. Don't try to predict what the teacher will present in each class. Treat each pose like it's your first time practicing it instead of just "going through the

motions." You are here for you, so give the practice (and your teacher) full attention.

11. *Respect yourself:* Do not compare yourself to others or what you think you should be able to do. Honor your limitations. Be patient and understanding with yourself. Listen to your breath and your body; this is a precious chance to deeply connect with your physical and mental states.

12. *Stay for the whole class: Savasana* (corpse pose) is practiced at the end of every class. You're selling yourself short, and disturbing all the other students, by leaving before class has ended (see Thing 23). If you find you don't enjoy a teacher's particular style, don't leave in the middle of the practice. Stay for the rest of the class and consider it a lesson well learned. Who knows—you may find a benefit to pushing beyond your comfort zone.

13. *Clean up before leaving:* The studio space should look just the way it did when you arrived, if not better. Make sure to replace all props you borrowed to their proper place and collect all of your belongings before departing. A sign of gratitude to the yoga teacher and studio staff is also warmly appreciated.

# — 12 —

# Keeping costs down

# − 12 −

# Keeping costs down

Sticker-shock alert! One yoga class can range from $10–$18. If you visit your favorite yoga studio three times a week, that's $120–$216 a month. Financial limitations are known to be one of the top reasons hundreds of thousands of people can't or don't practice yoga on a regular basis. As I mentioned at the very beginning of this book, nothing can stand in your way of practicing yoga. Here are effective ways to help overcome all those dollar signs.

## Buy class packages

Almost every yoga studio offers their students class passes in which a set of five to twenty classes is paid for at once. Those admissions are credited to your name, and you can use them over a certain amount of time (usually three to six months). Depending on the pass you buy, you can save $2–$7 per class!

Some studios also offer an introductory deal of three classes at a dramatically reduced price for new students. These passes must be redeemed within a very short time frame (often two weeks) but are a fantastic way to try a few different teachers at one studio for a low financial commitment.

## Community classes

Scan local yoga studio schedules for "community classes," which are offered at a lower per-class rate, usually occurring once or twice a week.

## Students, teachers, and seniors

Call yoga studios and ask if they offer discounts for local teachers, students, or senior citizens. Many do! You'll need to present an ID proving your claim, in turn saving you $2–$5 per class.

## Pay by donation

A new trend in yoga studios has emerged, with establishments all over the country offering some (or all) of their classes on a donation basis. You simply pay what you can, but the differences end there—all classes are still taught by certified teachers. If you can afford to pay $10–$15 per class then do so, but if you need to cut back one week, you can pay $5 for a while, increasing that amount when your finances improve.

## Volunteer exchange

Cleaning, organizing, checking students in for classes, answering e-mails—a yoga studio is a business like any other. They need help to keep their place running smoothly, and you may be just what they're looking for. Ask the manager of your local studio if they offer yoga classes in exchange for volunteer help. Mention any particular talents or formal experience you have (writing, graphic design, accounting), and your offer will seem all the more tantalizing.

## Other local outlets

A yoga studio isn't the only place to take yoga classes . . . but you knew that, right?

Have a gym membership? Check the class schedule. There's a very good chance the gym offers yoga classes that are included in your regular fee.

Have cable or satellite TV? Many providers offer free on-demand channels, with some including yoga classes. Check with your local TV provider for fitness-related programs or channels available.

Look into adult education programs offered by your local school system or nearby colleges. Weekly yoga classes of different levels may be available for a very affordable price, lasting six to eight weeks.

Most lululemon stores (check lululemon.com for locations) offer a free weekly sixty-minute yoga class, often on Saturday or Sunday. Check your local library or community center; many offer affordable yoga classes too.

## At-home helpers

Once you have a solid understanding of alignment, take advantage of all the benefits of practicing yoga at home. Countless DVDs, podcasts, and Web sites offer classes that are just like the ones you adore at the yoga studio. See Thing 24 for a list of all these money-saving resources.

## Embrace Yoga Day

Presented by the Yoga Alliance, Yoga Day USA is a one-day annual event when yoga studios across the country offer their classes or special workshops for free! Visit Yogadayusa.org for more details and to sign up for updates.

# — 13 —

# We are family

# ～ 13 ～

# We are family

Yoga is an intensely unique journey. What you may not know is that *asanas* (poses) aren't the only path to the mental, physical, and spiritual union that is "yoga." Although some people choose to follow only one path, they are all intimately intertwined. Think of the concept of yoga as a tree: the five different paths of yoga, discussed in the following paragraphs, are the roots to that tree. Without each one of them feeding the tree, it could not grow.

"The ocean refuses no river and all paths of yoga lead us to ourselves and ultimately, the divine within," says David Lurey. "We will all find different ways of self-explorations that feed our personal needs at that time—we must be open to that change.

Different stages of life will call forth different aspects of the practices of all these forms of yoga."

## *Hatha* (the path of physical discipline)

The ever-famous yoga postures fall into this category, along with *pranayama* (breathing techniques). Learning to control the body, its subtle life force—*prana*—and its senses is the ultimate goal. *Asanas* also strengthen the physical body to prepare it for long periods of meditation (see *Raja*).

## *Raja* (the path of mental discipline)

Often lumped together with *hatha* yoga, *raja* yoga is all about meditation, with the goal of mental control. During meditation, the wall between our minds and the rest of the spiritual, metaphysical world is slowly broken down. *Raja* and *hatha* yoga are often practiced as one yogic path, both working toward ultimate self-awareness.

## Karma (the path of selfless service or action)

Helping others without thinking of any possible success, honor, or rewards is the core of karma. Every time we interact with others is a chance to act from a pure, divine-like nature instead of from our human ego. Karma is directly related to the concept of cause and effect—all we do will have rippling repercussions for ourselves and others. Numerous yoga-related charities have been founded upon the concept of karma: GreenYoga. org, OffTheMatIntoTheWorld.org, YogaHope.org, TheArtOfYogaProject.org, Niroga.org, StreetYoga. org, YogaBehindBars.com, YogaForYouth.org, and LineageProject.org, just to name a few.

## *Bhakti* (the path of devotion or faith)

Being able to see the divine nature in all beings allows us to become more tolerant and accepting of the variety in our world. Whether you believe in

God, Jesus Christ, Buddha, Krishna, Muhammad, someone else, or no one at all, everyone can practice *bhakti*. Pure, selfless love for a person, concept, or religious being can involve prayer, chanting, mantras, rituals, or worship. The key element is a deep, unwavering emotional connection to our version of the divine, releasing our attachment to our own identity.

*Notable bhakti and karma yogis:* Mother Teresa, Martin Luther King, Jr., Gandhi. These individuals lived their lives in accordance with the concepts of *bhakti* and karma yoga.

## Jnana (the path of knowledge)

Using personal will to obtain wisdom amongst mounds of ignorance makes jnana one of the most difficult paths of yoga. Developing the mental and spiritual strength to concentrate and endure the conflicting opposites of nature requires a revolutionary shift in perception. Jnana is rarely practiced before the yogi becomes exceptionally experienced at all other paths of yoga, which provide vital lessons that prepare the body and mind.

*Notable jnana yogis:* Kabbalistic scholars, Jesuit priests, Benedictine monks.

# – 14 –

# More than *asanas*

# ~ 14 ~

# More than *asanas*

If the five yogic paths are the roots to the "tree" of yoga, then the eight limbs or steps from Patanjali's *Yoga Sutras* are its branches. Each limb must be tended to in order for the tree to remain healthy and vibrant. Compared to the eightfold path of Buddhism or the Ten Commandments of Christianity and Judaism, the eight limbs of yoga are a straightforward set of personal and ethical guidelines for living a conscious, meaningful life.

In the next seven tips, I'll discuss each limb of yoga in more detail. The first five limbs are known as the "outer practices" (*bahiranga*), and the last three limbs are known as the "inner practices" (*antaranga*). The outer practices are geared toward a more ethical, honorable lifestyle that separates us from our ego. The inner practices are more difficult, training our minds spiritually in order to connect with the divine energy in everyone and everything.

For now, let's cover the most common starting place for modern yogis: *asana*. Technically the third of the eight limbs of yoga, *asanas,* or postures, are a straightforward way of learning to stabilize the mind and body at the same time. Focusing on particular muscles, organs, or tendons in each yoga pose strengthens the body and releases stress while honing the mind for meditation. From Thing 13, you may recall that *hatha*, one of the five roots of yoga, is about *asanas* as well. *Hatha* also exemplifies how important it is to train the physical body to be strong and comfortable while the mind expands.

Little-known fact: yoga was originally developed to prepare monks and other spiritual practitioners for meditation. Often sitting still for hours at a time, their bodies would become stiff and achy, forcing them to move and lose concentration. By practicing yoga before meditation, they could remain exceptionally still for over eight hours!

"As early as the fourteenth century, sages were warning that if you practice *asanas* without the meditative aspect of yoga, the postures can actually become obstacles to liberation," says Frank Jude Boccio. "Without mindfulness, we can become attached to particular sensations and achievements. If we fixate on *asana*, then when things change through age or illness, we aren't capable of doing what we once could and then fall into despair. Authentic yoga is to frce oneself with identifying the body or mind as Self."

~ 15 ~

# *Yamas:* everyday ethics

# – 15 –

## *Yamas:* everyday ethics

The first two limbs of yoga are the moral guidelines, some of which may seem a bit obvious. The *yamas* [yuh-muhs] are the "don'ts" while the *niyamas* [nee-yuh-muh] (Thing 16) are the "dos," though that is a very simplified perspective. "In modern life, it is commonly accepted that *asana* practice leads to following the *yamas* and *niyamas*," says David Lurey. Following an ethical code is yet another way to train our minds to be disciplined, bringing awareness to the subtle differences within our bodies and minds. Establishing our own set of ethics reminds us that we are all naturally kind, honest, compassionate people. The five *yamas* are:

## 1. *Ahimsa* [uh-him-sah]

Translated as "nonharming" or "nonviolence." Show compassion for all creatures; this includes humans, animals, and plants. A lack of violence and cruelty is obvious, but it also means injecting understanding and kindness into every situation. Be cooperative and do no harm.

## 2. *Satya* [suht-yah]

Translated as "truthfulness" or "honesty," both in speech and thought. Sometimes, the truth hurts. Before we speak, we must consider the situation deeply. If being honest would be too painful to the other person, simply abstain from speaking. This isn't to say that the truth shouldn't be told—if someone is hurting others (whether human, plant, or animal), we must speak out. Avoid exaggeration, deceptions, or downright lying.

## 3. *Asteya* [as-tay-ya]

Translated as "nonstealing." Do not take advantage of anyone or anything. This applies to physically stealing things, but also emotions and private thoughts or secrets. If it was not freely given, it should not be taken. Everyone's time, energy, ideas, and independence are precious and, in a sense, divine. We should not demand things from others or forcefully monopolize them in any way.

## 4. *Brahmacharya* [brah-muh-chahr-yuh]

Translated as "continence" or "nonlust." Though celibacy is not required, we should abstain from meaningless sexual encounters and embrace monogamy. Forming relationships through truth and understanding should come far before adding the physical, passion-fueled element into the mix. By moderating how often we give our physical body to others, we do not take needlessly from others, fuel our ego's desires, or sacrifice our connection to our spiritual self.

## 5. *Aparigraha* [a-pa-ri-gra-ha]

Translated as "non-covetousness" or "non-possessiveness." Take or obtain no more than you need to live a safe and healthy life. We only deserve what we have earned—anything else is stealing or taking advantage of someone else. Yogic teachings interpret that hoarding, collecting, or being downright greedy shows a lack of faith that the divine will provide for us when we truly need it. Yes, we do need to work for a living, but our lives can still be complete without the latest house, car, clothes, electronic gadgets, or rare delicacies. Let go of attachments, both materially and emotionally, understanding that all is impermanent. Our ability to change with the times is one of our strongest skills.

It's easy to see why a yogic lifestyle is often associated with living sustainably and not consuming animal products. If we trip up and bend one of the guidelines of these *yamas,* the only punishment we face is from ourselves. We don't become "bad" people, but we have to suffer the consequences of our elected actions. "If we made *yamas* the central focus of our life, then we'd be living our yoga," says Frank Jude Boccio.

Want to be happy and healthy? Stop suffering and do the right thing. That can bring you much more happiness than temporary indulgences (your wallet may thank you too).

# – 16 –

# *Niyamas:* everyday actions

# – 16 –

# *Niyamas:* everyday actions

From how to treat others (*yamas*; see Thing 15) to how we treat ourselves, *niyamas* [nee-yuh-muh] is the second of the eight limbs of yoga. The *niyamas* are a natural extension and daily companion to the *yamas*. Another type of inner strength is derived from treating ourselves with responsibility and respect. These are the "rules" or "laws" we actively follow in relation to our own well-being and development. The five *niyamas* are:

## 1. *Sauca* [sow-cha]

Translated as "purity" or "cleanliness." It almost goes without saying that we should keep our physical body (inside and out), home, office, and yoga practice spaces clean and tidy. Additionally, we should seek to have a pure mind and intention in life. Cleansing ourselves of our internal poisons (chemical and emotional) through *asanas* (see Thing 14) and *pranayama* (see Thing 17), lends to purifying our spirit and moving forward with genuine purpose. Your body really is a temple.

## 2. *Santosa* [sun-toe-shuh]

Translated as "contentment" or "satisfaction." True happiness has nothing to do with external circumstances. We can be at peace any day, any time, anywhere, with anyone. Each moment offers us something to appreciate and something else to learn. Everything happens for a reason (another example of karma), so move through life with humility and modesty. We are where we are because of our own actions. Accept the truth, what life has handed you, and keep growing. Enjoy what you do have instead of regretting what or who you don't possess.

### 3. *Tapas* [tuhp-uhs]

Translated as "discipline" or "austerity." Consistency is a key element of growing physically, mentally, emotionally, and spiritually. We get what we give, and the more we put into our yoga practice, the more it will positively impact all areas of our lives. As we've learned, yoga isn't just physical poses, though they are an important element (as are good posture and strong muscles). We must also practice using our energy in a disciplined way through what we say, think, eat, and do, with the aim of achieving control over the body and mind to prepare ourselves for a more spiritual purpose.

### 4. *Svadhyaya* [svuhd-hyu-yuh]

Translated as "self-study" or "spiritual study." We should seek to educate ourselves in two ways. First, studying spiritual texts helps to promote a better understanding of the miracles of life and all its possibilities. Second, we must study through personal contemplation, often done through meditation (see Thing 19). We can't connect with the divine energy in us until we find it within ourselves. Learn your limitations, accept past mistakes, forgive others' indiscretions against you, and remove the self-destructive habits that keep you from blossoming.

## 5. *Isvarapranidhana* [ish-vuhru-pruhnid-hunuh]

Translated as "devotion." Before you get worried, no one is going to force you to believe in God, or Buddha, or anyone else. In the final *niyama,* we learn we must let go of the belief that we can control everything. There is a scientifically unexplainable omnipresent energy that connects us all and transcends the temporary things in life. So surrender to the spiritual force in your life. Be able to part with any of your difficulties, possessions, or accomplishments, for they are all temporary.

## ~ 17 ~

# *Pranayama:* nothing beats a good breath

# ⁓ 17 ⁓

# *Pranayama:* nothing beats a good breath

W hen you get flustered, you're probably reminded to take a deep breath. That's great advice! The fourth limb of yoga is all about breathing. Yet another way to strengthen the body and expand the mind, yogic breathing techniques help us control the flow of *prana,* our vital internal energy that flows like a constant air current. "Yoga without the breath is like a thunderstorm without lightning: you need to have the breath before you can feel the true power of any *asana,*" says Peter Guinosso.

Any type or amount of stress can cause our sympathetic nervous system to kick in, triggering our unconscious fight-or-flight response. Conscious, controlled breathing helps our parasympathetic nervous system to take over, allowing our brain waves to slow down, quieting the body and mind. From here, we can approach life's difficulties with balanced intelligence, instead of split-second emotions.

When angry, nervous, or confused, you will likely notice that your breathing becomes very shallow, barely filling up your lungs. Additionally, your muscles are likely to tighten in your shoulders, neck, back, or stomach. On the other hand, sleeping babies can be seen breathing deeply from their bellies. The powerful connection between the body, mind, and emotions is why *pranayama* [prah-nuh-yuh-muh] techniques are taught side-by-side with *asanas* in regular yoga practice.

An obviously natural body function, breathing requires intentional focus to break the action down into four steps: inhalation (*puraka*), retention (*kumbhaka*), exhalation (*rechaka*), and respite (*shunyaka*). Though there are many *pranayama* methods, I'd like to share one of the most basic with you. Called *sukha purvaka pranayama* ("the easy breath that precedes all others"), this four-part technique helped me through everyday stressors, severe depression, and panic attacks.

1. Sit comfortably on the floor or in a chair, eyes closed and spine straight.

2. Breathe naturally for a few minutes, releasing bodily tension and mental distractions.

3. Through your nose only, complete the following sequence of actions:
- Inhale slowly into your belly for six counts/ seconds.
- Hold the breath inside for six counts/seconds.
- Exhale slowly and evenly for six counts/ seconds.
- Pause for six counts/seconds.

4. Repeat the sequence three to eight times.

This can be done anywhere and anytime, and those around are none the wiser. I find it especially useful in meetings, traffic, and before eating. "In any interaction or conversation, to place your attention in your heart using your deep, attentive breathing brings about a state of receptivity [and] more appropriate responses and diminishes reactivity," says Elena Brower, founder of Virayoga studio in New York. "These are qualities of good listeners—trustworthy, patient, inspiring people who are wonderful to be around."

## – 18 –

## *Pratyahara:*
## withdrawing the senses

# − 18 −

## *Pratyahara:* withdrawing the senses

The fifth limb of yoga teaches us to remove the influence the outside world has on us. Sight, smell, taste, touch, hearing—all five of our main senses are bombarded with stimuli on an enormous scale. Developing non-attachment to our worldly sensations, we can learn that our consciousness isn't found solely in our senses. When undistracted by outside images and items, scents, flavors, textures, and noises, your body can truly be still while your mind expands. "We practice keeping all sense doors open; the 'trick' is to learn to do so without getting caught in the sensorial experience," says Frank Jude Boccio.

From your yoga mat and meditation cushion to your morning commute and weekly business meetings, *pratyahara* [pruh-tyah-hah-ruh] is another element of yoga that you can practice anywhere, anytime. Like all people, places, and things continually change, our sensory experiences change each and every moment. Everything in life is not permanent. "Modern yogis are asked to do something incredibly challenging: to be good people in a world that is full of temptation and opportunities to act irresponsibly," says David Lurey. By quieting our rapid-fire minds and turning inward, we can connect with the everlasting part of ourselves (often referred to as the soul).

As you master *pratyahara*, you will be able to genuinely focus on the importance of the moment without becoming attached to it. *Pratyahara* is why most people are more at peace in the countryside than in a bustling city. With fewer stimuli bombarding your senses, you are able to feel, heal, and grow your pure nature (a key goal with meditation). From here, we can objectively interpret our impulses, cravings, and reactions of our world. This particular limb of yoga is also a significant transition from the externally focused limbs already discussed (*yamas, niyamas, asana, pranayama*), and the upcoming internally focused limbs (*dharana, dhyana, samadhi*).

# – 19 –

## *Dharana:*
## cultivating concentration

# – 19 –

# *Dharana:*
# cultivating concentration

After learning to control our senses with *pratyahara* (see Thing 18), the sixth limb of yoga hones our mental focus. Now and then, we're all guilty of a scattered mentality and disorganized thoughts. Concentrating on a sole object, person, or task is extremely difficult; just thinking about it gives me a headache. Giving into the flighty nature of our minds only leads to trouble. A solid, progressive practice can help us take control of the physical vessel we've been blessed (and cursed) with.

*Dharana* is often taught alongside meditation, which it also prepares us for. You may have heard someone say, "Just clear your mind." That's not helpful. Yes, we do want to remove thoughts, fears, and distractions, but let's start simpler. Instead, we must first learn to focus all our mental energy on one thing.

Whether a picture, mantra, or random entity, this one thing shouldn't hold much emotional connection, for that will cause distractions. Try focusing on just a simple object. How about a pencil? Or sand? Maybe a glass of water or the flame of a candle? Just keep the image in your mind. If something else comes in, just let it go right back out. Focus on your object while seated, breathing in a natural, calm way through your nose. Keep your face and entire body calm with no physical tension. Start with two to five minutes of *dharana* each day. When you find that easy, increase the time.

"When we focus the mind to a single point, it is like the honey dripping from a dropper—no splash or diversion, just a clean, simple strand of consciousness," says David Lurey. Soon, you'll be able to fully concentrate on any conversation, quandary, or passing moment. Like any other part of yoga, only practice will increase your aptitude. Next, we'll use the precise concentration we've learned to enter a true state of meditation.

# – 20 –

# *Dhyana:* meditating

# — 20 —

## *Dhyana:* meditating

Our consistent practice of *dharana* (Thing 19)
will eventually lead us to *dhyana*, a true state
of meditation. Contrary to common perception, you
can't just sit down, close your eyes, and "meditate."
However, you can sit with eyes closed, focusing on
one thing and working toward the mental state of
meditation.

Before I confuse you further, let me define meditation. Meditation is the constant observation of the
mind from a logical, emotionally neutral standpoint.
"Meditation is yoga; it's not something you 'do,'"
says Frank Jude Boccio. "Most of the techniques
taught as meditation are simply devices that help
cultivate *dhyana*." All six limbs of yoga that come
before *dhyana* have helped prepare for this state of

true meditation. From that perspective, you can see that true meditation can't be obtained without considerable effort—but it is more than worth it.

Meditation's objective view of ourselves allows the mind to grow immensely, which in turn connects us to the wide expanse of the rest of the universe. Meditating is by no means easy, boring, or just another thing on your to-do list. When we pass from practicing *dharana* to experiencing *dhyana,* we struggle to put the moment into words. The realization that what we perceive as reality is nothing but a farce often accompanies achieving *dhyana.* Our bodies are nothing more than vessels that hold our everlasting spirits. Meditation helps you transcend from human existence to something otherworldly.

"Have I experienced meditation?" Unless you've been practicing for years, probably not, but the opportunity to experience it is always available. If your mind is aware of any distraction, then you are still practicing *dharana.* Do not merely seek *dhyana,* but seek it as a stepping stone to something even better.

The journey is never over, as our last limb of yoga will show.

# *Samadhi:* becoming balanced

# – 21 –

## *Samadhi:* becoming balanced

Whether you call it nirvana, enlightenment, ecstasy, satori, or *samadhi* ("equal thinking"), the eighth limb of yoga is the culmination of all our physical and mental hard work. As with the sixth and seventh limbs of yoga, the final stage of true yoga is difficult to put into words. The experience speaks for itself.

Upon reaching *samadhi* [suh-mah-dee], the senses become completely still while the heart and mind combine with the spirit of the universe. This is a state of true bliss that cannot be fathomed without encountering it firsthand. Our day-to-day occurrences take on a whole new meaning when we have become "superconscious" or "extra-sensory." It is the ultimate level of non-attachment, in which one lives in a state of peaceful contemplation, heightened awareness, and expansive compassion. This is the true definition of yoga (see Thing 1). "*Samadhi* is not the goal of yoga—it is merely a door to liberation," says Frank Jude Boccio.

In order to reach *samadhi*, we must practice the full eight limbs of yoga on a daily basis. However, that's not to say we should jump into doing them all at once. The first five limbs of yoga can be easily practiced concurrently. The last three limbs of yoga are a bit more progressive, focused strictly on state-of-mind. No matter your schedule, budget, or location, yoga is meant to be practiced every minute of every day. "Discipline is the true key to freedom," says David Lurey. "Discipline is what gives a yogi direction as well as benchmarks for development and growth."

A physical yoga practice is just as important as all the other elements of yoga. It may be hard to imagine meeting yourself on your yoga mat every day, but that is what needs to be done. This doesn't mean you have to practice ninety minutes every day at the same time or same location. You don't have to take a yoga class every day for the rest of your life—you can imagine how expensive that would be! For just ten minutes each morning or evening, listen to your body while practicing poses that remove strain and enhance strength. This will prepare your mind and spirit for all the other limbs of yoga.

Just like committing to a healthier diet or learning a new hobby, a little bit of yoga every day can make all the difference. You owe it to yourself to visit that new yoga studio, rent that yoga DVD, or invest in a high-quality yoga mat. This is your health, your consciousness, your chance to grow. I hope I have opened a new door for you. It's time to walk on through.

# – 22 –

# Coming into the light

# — 22 —

# Coming into the light

One of the most well-known yoga sequences, *surya namaskar* ("sun salutation") has numerous physical and spiritual benefits. By completing the eight postures in a twelve-step flowing sequence, the body's muscles become limber while the body also burns calories. You begin to feel the distinct warmth and clarity of the sun both internally and externally, thanks to increased blood flow and *prana*. Traditionally performed at the beginning of the day, *surya namaskar* can be an invigorating full-yoga practice anytime, anywhere.

Praising the sun, whether religiously or simply for its usefulness, has been happening for tens of thousands of years. The sun regulates our sleep schedules, marks changes of the seasons, and helps our food grow, among many other things. How old the *surya namaskar* sequence is has been highly debated. In modern terms, this series of poses is often seen as an appreciative gesture for the physical light and personal insight the sun provides.

As with all yoga poses, your movements are connected to your breath: exhale when you fold or contract, inhale when you stretch or extend. Also, each move should be executed with the utmost awareness; no yoga practice should be performed sloppily—this is a moving meditation. For beginners, it is recommended you complete only five rounds of *surya namaskar,* later progressing to ten to fifteen at the start of every practice.

1. Stand tall at the front of your yoga mat, feet together, arms at your sides, eyes closed. Bring your hands together in a prayer-like position in front of your chest. Exhale.

2. Inhale while opening your eyes and sweeping your arms directly above your head, then reconnecting your palms and looking up at your hands.

3. Exhale as you bend down over your strong legs, bending your knees slightly if this feels too uncomfortable. Try to place your hands or fingertips on either side of your feet.

4. Bend over far enough for your hands to fully reach the ground on either side of your feet. Inhale and step one foot back into a lunge-like pose, placing your hands on both sides of your front foot. Curve your back slightly, bend your knees if there is too much strain in the backs of your legs, and look straight ahead.

5. Exhale and step your other leg back into a plank position, with your spine in a straight line (most folks need to raise their buttocks more). Inhale while

still in this pose, with your weight evenly distributed among your arms (by pushing strong against the floor), legs (by pushing your heels away from you), and abs (tighten 'em up!).

6. Exhale and lower your whole body straight down to the floor as though doing a push-up. If this is too difficult (I can barely do it!), lower your knees to the ground first, then your chest, followed by your forehead. Your hips should still be in the air, having no contact with the floor, and the bottom of your toes still in contact with the mat.

7. Inhale as you fold the tops of your toes flat on the mat while straightening your legs, pushing your body slightly forward. With your hands still on the mat, push off the ground with your arms straight, bending your upper body slightly backward. Keep your legs strong and lifted, with only your hands and toes coming into contact with the mat.

8. Exhale as you curl the bottom of your feet back into contact with the mat, pressing down with your heels, lifting your hips into the sky while keeping your arms straight. Pressing your hands into the mat, put most of your weight on the area between your thumb and forefinger, helping to release strain in your shoulders and upper back.

9. Inhale as you bring one foot forward (the same foot you stepped back with in number four) again into a lunge, keeping your chest lifted, eyes straight ahead, and hands on opposite sides of your front foot.

10. Exhale as you step your other foot forward, bringing your feet together and lifting your hips up into the air, folding over your standing legs.

11. Inhale as you raise your straight back up to standing, sweeping your arms from your sides to straight overhead, bringing palms together and looking up at your joined hands.

12. Exhale as you slowly lower your arms to your sides, looking straight ahead.

For each round, use the same foot you step back with in number four to step forward with in number nine, alternating each round (e.g., round one: left foot back, left foot forward; round two: right foot back, right foot forward).

# ~ 23 ~

# Understanding the significance of *savasana*

## – 23 –

# Understanding the significance of
# *savasana*

The final pose of every yoga class and personal practice is *savasana* (corpse pose), and for very good cause. You're not just "lying on the floor, doing nothing." This is a time of relaxation, for both the body and the mind. *Savasana* can actually prove to be the toughest yoga pose of all: with your body still, your mind is free to wander, sometimes stirring up past regrets, current fears, and future uncertainties. Allowing yourself to acknowledge your thoughts but not be emotionally consumed by them is the first step toward a true meditative state (see Things 19 and 20). Unlike meditation, though, you are not trying to focus on one specific thing. *Savasana* is just about relaxation, no matter your mental patterns. "*Savasana* embraces the misunderstood concept of 'doing nothing'—and we get to realize there is power in it," says Jeanie Garden. Of course, you have to stay awake too.

Our modern, hectic lives are crying out for daily *savasana*. A testament to this desire are the pose's wide-reaching benefits:

- Relaxing the body's muscles and organ systems
- Reducing issues with fatigue, headache, and insomnia
- Relieving stress, depression, and anxiety while calming the mind
- Possibly helping to lower blood pressure

Leaving yoga class before *savasana* is not only extremely rude (see Thing 11), but you're also cheating yourself and those around you from experiencing its therapeutic benefits. When you practice yoga at home, *savasana* is your ever-important peaceful time to yourself. This relaxation time allows your body to process everything it has been put through during your yoga practice. Skip it and it's like you never even stepped onto your mat. "Everything comes together in *savasana,* and when you skip it or shortchange it, you miss out on a tremendous opportunity to absorb and consolidate the benefits of your practice," says Natasha Rizopoulos.

As the name implies, during corpse pose, you lie on your back, arms relaxed at your sides, palms up, legs extended and spread apart two to six inches with feet rolled out the sides. You body temperature will drop while in *savasana,* which can be very distracting, so I recommend covering up with a blanket. For extra comfort, you can place a bolster under your knees, a pillow under your head, and an eye pillow over your eyes. Mentally check in with every part of your body, ensuring it is not holding any extra tension. Be sure that your head doesn't roll too far back or forward (very bad for your neck), keeping your chin parallel to the floor.

The average recommendation is five minutes of *savasana* for every thirty minutes of the rest of your physical yoga practice. Start with five minutes and work up to ten, fifteen, or even thirty minutes, depending on what your body needs.

# – 24 –
# Putting it into practice

# — 24 —

# Putting it into practice

Enough *about* yoga—let's *do* yoga! Whether you are looking for a local yoga studio, are ready to begin an at-home practice, or need to take your yoga on the road, I'll help you find just what you need.

## Find local classes

The easiest way to find great local classes is to ask others. Yoga practitioners will happily tell you about the great studios they frequent, along with their favorite instructors. Alternatively, you can visit YogaAlliance.org and search for yoga studios in your area ("Registered Schools"). *Yoga Journal* magazine also maintains a directory of yoga classes at Yoga Journal.com/Directory. Of course, a Google.com search of "yoga studio, [your location]" will draw up results as well. Last but not least, check with your local public education system, community center, or community college. Nearly all of them offer once-a-week yoga classes, often presented in six- to eight-week packages.

## DVDs

The collection of available yoga DVDs has expanded exponentially in the past decade. From beginner to advanced, children to seniors, vinyasa flow to restorative, there's a DVD for everyone. Also, ask your friends and family about their favorite yoga DVDs. You can't do better than a personal recommendation. Not ready to buy? Visit your local library; many have fitness DVDs available for rent. Many local yoga studios also sell DVDs; ask your yoga teacher or someone else who works at the studio for suggestions. Here are some of the most popular online outlets for yoga DVDs:

YogaJournal.com/Shop
Gaiam.com ("Media Library")
AcaciaCatalog.com ("Fitness")
BodyWisdomMedia.com
WhiteLotus.org ("Books and DVDs")
RaviAna.com ("Yoga Store")
YogaKids.com ("Store")
ViniYoga.com ("What We Offer" then "Products")
OmYoga.com ("Shop")
BeeTwixt.com [teens only]
YogaMinded.com [teens only]
AgelessYoga.org [seniors only]
LiliasYoga.com [seniors only]

## Music CDs (for yoga practice or meditation)

Listening to music while practicing yoga can help you stay motivated and open-minded. During meditation, music can help your mind elevate and expand in all directions. For your yoga practice, any music can suffice; some prefer to stick with more traditional rhythms and chanting, while others listen to hip-hop, reggae, jazz, or rock. A large variety of tunes during meditation isn't recommended; it can cause your mind to fly in too many directions at once. Instead, pick an instrumental mix to let your mind bloom. As with DVDs, many local yoga studios also sell music CDs, so be sure to check out their offerings. Here are few great online outlets for music and meditation CDs:

SoundsTrue.com
NuToneMusic.com
ModernMeditations.com
KrishnaDasMusic.com
WhiteSwanRecords.com
YogaJournal.com ("Multimedia" for free downloads)

## Online Classes

Ready for the next big thing in yoga? I'm talking about online yoga classes. There are a few obvious benefits and drawbacks, similar to those of DVDs. Pros: yoga practices led by established pros, portability, and affordability. Cons: no personal adjustments, no community vibe. No matter your preferences, Web-based video yoga classes are a fun supplement to your regular routine. Here are a few of my favorite sources for online yoga classes, many of which can be downloaded to your computer or MP3 video player (perfect for traveling):

YogaToday.com
YogaYak.com
YogaJournal.com/Video
YogaJournal.com ("Practice" then "Practice Downloads")
YogaWithLes.com/Videos/
MyYogaOnline.com
Yo-Fi.com
YogaGlo.com
CorePowerYoga.com ("Yoga on Demand")
GaiamYogaClub.com

*Note:* Yes, some do require a one-time or monthly membership. Only you can decide if the investment is worth it for you and your situation.

# — 25 —

# Taking a getaway

# ‒ 25 ‒

## Taking a getaway

We all need a break from the daily grind, but not from our yoga. When you're ready to skip town, make sure to grab your mat because now more than ever, yoga has become a key element in a growing number of vacation resorts, retreats, festivals, and conferences. These are also great opportunities to step outside of your comfort zone, trying a yoga style or teacher you wouldn't normally pursue.

"If we take some time and experience on a retreat, we can weave that into our life at home," says Les Leventhal. "Our inner and outer worlds are calmer and at ease, then those benefits spread to other folks in our lives." Whether a getaway for one person, couple, family, or group of 30,000, yoga will make your travels infinitely more memorable.

## Vacations and retreats

Countless hotels, spas, and retreat destinations offer yoga as part of their services. If you already have a location in mind, the easiest thing to do is hunt down hotels and inquire about yoga classes or local yoga studios. Alternatively, visit YogaJournal.com/Directory and search under the "Vacations and Retreats" category for options all over the world. A Google.com search for yoga vacations or retreats will often turn up numerous results, but be sure to ask lots of questions before you book, as this is the travel industry and scams do still exist. Last but not least, you may need to look no further than your local yoga studio. Many larger establishments arrange their own regional or international vacations. Also talk to your favorite teacher about any upcoming events or getaways she may have planned.

## Festivals and conferences

If vacations are meant to be peaceful and introspective, yoga festivals and conferences are the exact opposite. This is your chance to interact with the larger yoga community and have some major fun. These events vary widely and often include an expansive list of activities: group lectures and yoga classes with well-known teachers, meditation, live music, fresh local food, evening dance parties, art galleries, local vendors, camping, and so much more. Festivals and conferences can be big shindigs of over 50,000 people or an intimate get-together of less than 2,000. Browse these Web sites for more details about just some of the spectacular yoga festivals and conferences held regularly:

YJEvents.com (nationwide)
YogaDayUSA.org (nationwide)
MidwestYoga.com (Illinois)
3HO.org (New Mexico and Florida)

TellurideYogaFestival.com (Colorado)
FlagstaffYogaFestival.com (Arizona)
WanderlustFestival.com (California)
YogaRocks.info (Colorado)
Eomega.org/omega/beingyoga (New York)
PendletonYogaRoundUp.com (Oregon)
EvolveFest.rog (New Jersey)
BhaktiFest.com (California)
VermontYogaFestival.com (Vermont)
WorldPeaceYogaConference.com (Ohio)
SacredThread.net (California)

# – 26 –

# Becoming a yoga pro

# – 26 –

# Becoming a yoga pro

Whether you are on the hunt for a new career or simply want to take your own practice to another level, a teacher training program may be what you are looking for. In yoga teacher training, you will delve boundlessly deeper into the traditions, scriptures, alignment, and applications of yoga. Location, time commitment, and prices vary widely, so before you decide to take this major step, do your research.

First, you need to decide what yoga style you would like to study. By now, you should have been personally practicing yoga for at least two years on a consistent basis (at least five days a week). This time frame includes classes at yoga studios, vacations, and in your own home. Consistency is vital because your personal experience will sustain your pledge to study further. At this point, you've likely identified which yoga style (or styles) you feel most comfortable with.

Next, it's time to pick out possible teacher training programs. Start local by inquiring whether your favorite local yoga studio offers a teacher training program. To expand your search, visit YogaJournal.com/Directory (under Category, select "Teacher Training and Workshops") and YogaAlliance.org/School_Search.cfm to find local, regional, national, and international teacher training possibilities.

The Yoga Alliance is a nonprofit that is seen as a major force in yoga teaching regulation. A 200-hour certification from Yoga Alliance is what many yoga studios and gyms look for when hiring new teachers. Make sure that the teacher programs you are interested in are approved by the Yoga Alliance; otherwise, you won't be able to get your training certification or the new title of Registered Yoga Teacher (RYT). Even if you are only studying to expand your own practice, Yoga Alliance–approved programs are established, diverse, and easily the best choice for fruitful knowledge.

Third, the legwork begins. It's time to send e-mails, make phone calls, and visit these schools in person, especially if you have never practiced there before. Teacher training programs can cost anywhere from $1,500 to $5,000 and last one to two months (meeting every day) or six months to an entire year (meeting on evenings, weekends, or extended visits). This is nothing short of a commitment and should be taken as seriously as buying a car or a house. The Yoga Alliance provides an excellent list of questions to use when analyzing teacher training courses, available at YogaAlliance.org/School_Search.cfm (click on "Choosing a Yoga School" at top-left).

I don't want to burst your bubble, but if you are considering becoming a yoga teacher, there are a few things you need to know. A yoga teacher is just like most writers, illustrators, and actors—you are a freelancer. Therefore, you have to pay for your own retirement fund, taxes, health care, liability insurance (e.g., YogaJournal.com/BenefitsPlus/), and more. That's the reality for anyone who is self-employed or starts their own business. Even teaching at a yoga studio or gym, you are not an employee of those locations. You are your own business, which can be exhilarating and stressful at the same time. This will be a definite change in your lifestyle, but taking your career into your own hands makes it an incomparable opportunity.

For some extra reading about the world of teaching training and yoga instruction, check out these resources:

- YogaJournal.com/For_Teachers
- *Teaching Yoga: Exploring the Teacher-Student Relationship* by Donna Farhi
- *Guiding Yoga's Light: Lessons for Yoga Teachers* by Nancy Gerstein

# ~ 27 ~

# Reading on

# ─ 27 ─

# Reading on

I'm sad to say that our journey together has ended. I hope that this book has inspired you to begin a beautiful yoga journey all on your own. As I mentioned in the Introduction, this book is just a drop in the vast ocean of available yoga knowledge. To help you continue on your path, I've created a list of some of my favorite yoga books, magazines, Web sites, and blogs. The world of yoga continues to expand and evolve, and these other outlets will help you stay in touch with those changes, your practice, and yourself. *Namaste* and many happy *asanas* ahead.

## Books (arranged according to aspects of yoga)

*Yoga: The Greater Tradition* by Dr. David Frawley
*The Yoga Sutra of Patanjali* by Edwin F. Bryant
*The Wisdom of Yoga* by Stephen Cope
*Hatha Yoga Pradipika* by Swami Muktibodhananda
*Bhagavad Gita: A New Translation* by Stephen Mitchell
*1,001 Pearls of Yoga Wisdom* by Liz Lark
*Yoga as Medicine* by Timothy B. McCall, M.D.
*30 Essential Poses* by Judith Hanson Lasater
*OM Yoga: A Guide to Daily Practice* by Cyndi Lee
*The Woman's Yoga Book* by Bobby Clennell
*Breathe: Yoga for Teens* by Mary Kaye Chryssicas
*Lilias! Yoga Gets Better with Age* by Lilias Folan
*The New Yoga for Healthy Aging* by Suza Francina
*Light on Yoga* by B. K. S. Iyengar
*Yoga Anatomy* by Leslie Kaminoff
*Mindfulness Yoga: The Awakened Union of Breath, Body, and Mind* by Frank Jude Boccio
*Living Your Yoga* by Judith Hanson Lasater
*Green Yoga* by Georg and Brenda Feuerstein

## Magazines

*Yoga Journal* (YogaJournal.com)
*Yoga+* (HimalayanInstitute.org/YogaPlus/)
*YOGA Magazine* (YogaMagazine.us)
*Yogi Times* (YogiTimes.com)
*LA Yoga* (LAYogaMagazine.com)
*NY Yoga* (NYYogaMagazine.com)
*Yoga Chicago* (YogaChicago.com)
*Ascent* (AscentMagazine.com; no longer published, but back issues still available)

## Web sites and blogs

Cyndisphere.com
Discover-Yoga-Online.com
ItsAllAboutYoga.com
ItsAllYogaBaby.com
Padmaease.Wordpress.com
YogaDeals.Blogspot.com

YogaDork.com
YogaInMySchool.com
YogaMovement.com

**Featured yoga teachers**

Frank Jude Boccio: MindfulnessYoga.net
Elena Brower: Virayoga.com
Les Leventhal: YogaWithLes.com
David Lurey: FindBalance.net
Jeanie Garden: JeanieYoga.com
Peter Guinosso: YogaIsLife.net
Natasha Rizopoulos: NatashaRizopoulos.com